For permission requests, write to the author at
Chachachandca@gmail.com

ISBN: 9798861634168

Varicose eczema Complete treatment

Varicose eczema

Complete treatment

BY TAYLOR JONES

Acknowledgment

We would like to express our sincere gratitude to all those who contributed to the creation of this comprehensive guide on Varicose Eczema.

First and foremost, we extend our appreciation to the healthcare professionals and experts in dermatology and vascular medicine whose invaluable knowledge and insights have enriched the content of this resource.

We are also thankful for the individuals who shared their personal experiences and stories, shedding light on the challenges of living with Varicose Eczema and the importance of raising awareness about this condition.

Furthermore, we acknowledge the dedicated team of researchers and writers who diligently compiled and organized the information presented here, ensuring its accuracy and clarity.

Finally, we want to thank our readers for their interest in learning more about Varicose Eczema. Our hope is that this guide will serve as a valuable source of information and support

Varicose eczema Complete treatment

for those affected by this condition and those seeking to understand it better.

Thank you all for your contributions and commitment to promoting health and well-being.

Introduction 6

Chapter 1 8

What is Varicose Eczema 8

Causes and Risk Factors 9

Chapter 2 11

symptoms of Varicose Eczema..11

Skin Changes 11

Potential Complications 13

Chapter 3 15

Diagnosis 15

Medical History and Physical Examination 15

Doppler Ultrasound 16

Other Diagnostic Tests 17

Varicose eczema Complete treatment

Chapter 4 18

Treatment Options...18

Lifestyle Changes 19

Topical Medications 20

Compression Therapy 20

Medications 21

Procedures and Surgery 21

Chapter 5 23

Prevention and Self-Care 23

Maintaining Healthy Leg Circulation 23

Skin Care Tips 24

Lifestyle Modifications 25

Chapter 6 26

Living with Varicose Eczema 26

Coping with Symptoms 27

Monitoring and Follow-up 28

Support and Resources 29

Varicose eczema Complete treatment

Conclusion 30

Summary of Varicose Eczema 30

Importance of Early Detection and Management 31

Varicose eczema Complete treatment

INTRODUCTION

Varicose eczema, often referred to as stasis dermatitis, is a skin condition that occurs in individuals with underlying circulatory problems, primarily in the lower extremities. This condition is a testament to the intricate connection between our vascular system and the health of our skin. While it may seem like an isolated dermatological issue, Varicose eczema is, in fact, a manifestation of an underlying vascular insufficiency that demands our attention.

At its core, Varicose eczema is the result of chronic venous insufficiency, a condition where the veins in the legs struggle to efficiently return blood to the heart. This leads to a buildup of pressure in the veins, causing them to become enlarged and tortuous, commonly known as varicose veins. As the veins struggle with this increased pressure, they can leak fluid and blood cells into the surrounding tissue. This leakage can trigger a cascade of events within the skin, leading to the development of Varicose eczema.

Varicose eczema Complete treatment

The hallmark of Varicose eczema is not only its distinctive appearance but also the array of uncomfortable symptoms it brings. The skin in affected areas becomes discolored, often taking on a reddish-brown or purplish hue. It may feel warm to the touch and is frequently accompanied by intense itching and discomfort. Left untreated, Varicose eczema can progress, potentially leading to complications such as skin ulcers and infections.

While Varicose eczema can be a persistent and bothersome condition, it is not without hope. Advances in medical understanding and treatment options have paved the way for effective management and relief. Through lifestyle modifications, topical treatments, compression therapy, and, in some cases, medical procedures, individuals can find relief from the symptoms and prevent further complications.

In this comprehensive guide on Varicose eczema, we will explore the various aspects of this condition, from its causes and symptoms to diagnosis, treatment options, and prevention strategies. Our aim is to provide you with a thorough understanding of Varicose eczema so that you can take proactive steps towards managing it and improving your quality

Varicose eczema Complete treatment

of life. Whether you are someone experiencing Varicose eczema or seeking to enhance your knowledge of this condition, we hope that this resource serves as a valuable source of information and support.

CHAPTER 1

WHAT IS VARICOSE ECZEMA

Varicose eczema, also known as stasis dermatitis, is a chronic skin condition that primarily affects the lower legs, ankles, and feet. It is closely associated with underlying circulatory problems, particularly chronic venous insufficiency. Unlike typical eczema, which is primarily driven by allergic reactions or genetic factors, Varicose eczema is a secondary skin condition caused by poor blood circulation in the veins of the lower extremities.

The development of Varicose eczema is a multi-step process. It typically begins with venous insufficiency, where the valves in

Varicose eczema Complete treatment

the leg veins fail to function correctly. This causes blood to pool in the veins, increasing pressure within them. As a result, the veins become enlarged and twisted, forming varicose veins. The increased pressure and fluid leakage from these veins can damage the surrounding tissues, including the skin.

The characteristic symptoms of Varicose eczema include

- Skin discoloration: The affected skin often takes on a reddish-brown or purplish hue due to the accumulation of blood cells and breakdown products in the tissue.

Itching: Intense itching is a common symptom of Varicose eczema, which can be quite distressing for individuals with this condition.

Varicose eczema Complete treatment

Dry and scaly skin: The skin in the affected area may become dry, scaly, and flaky.

Swelling: Swelling, medically known as edema, can occur as fluid accumulates in the affected tissues.

Skin changes: Over time, the skin may thicken and harden, and it can become more vulnerable to injury.

CAUSES AND RISK FACTORS

The primary cause of Varicose eczema is chronic venous insufficiency, but several risk factors and contributing factors can increase the likelihood of developing this condition. Understanding these factors is essential for both prevention and management. Here are some key causes and risk factors associated with Varicose eczema:

Venous insufficiency: As mentioned earlier, the failure of valves in the leg veins to prevent backward flow of blood is the central cause. This leads to varicose veins, which can trigger Varicose eczema.

Varicose eczema Complete treatment

Age: Varicose eczema is more common in older adults because vein function tends to weaken with age.

Gender: Women are more susceptible to this condition, possibly due to hormonal changes and the pressure exerted on leg veins during pregnancy.

Obesity: Excess body weight can increase the pressure on leg veins, exacerbating venous insufficiency.

Family history: A genetic predisposition to weak vein valves can increase the risk.

Prolonged standing or sitting: Occupations or lifestyles that involve extended periods of sitting or standing can contribute to poor circulation, increasing the risk of Varicose eczema.

Previous blood clots: A history of deep vein thrombosis DVT or other vascular issues can damage vein valves and increase the risk.

Trauma or injury: Direct injury to the legs or surgical procedures can damage veins and lead to venous insufficiency.

Smoking: Smoking can harm blood vessels and exacerbate circulation problems.

Varicose eczema Complete treatment

Understanding these causes and risk factors is crucial for early detection and management of Varicose eczema. Identifying and addressing the underlying circulatory issues is a key component of effective treatment and prevention strategies.

CHAPTER 2

SYMPTOMS OF VARICOSE ECZEMA

Skin Changes

One of the hallmark symptoms of Varicose Eczema is noticeable changes in the skin's appearance, particularly in the lower legs and ankles. These changes are a result of the underlying venous insufficiency and the subsequent effects on the skin's microcirculation. Skin changes associated with Varicose Eczema may include:

Varicose eczema Complete treatment

Discoloration: The affected skin often takes on a reddish-brown or purplish hue due to the accumulation of red blood cells and breakdown products in the tissue. This discoloration is known as hemosiderin staining.

Hyperpigmentation: Over time, the skin in the affected area can become darker than the surrounding skin. This is due to the chronic inflammation and increased melanin production.

Thickened skin: The skin may thicken and harden, a condition referred to as lichenification. This occurs as a response to chronic irritation and inflammation.

Scaling and flakiness: Dry, scaly patches may develop on the skin's surface, leading to itching and discomfort.

Itching and Discomfort:

Itching and discomfort are common and often distressing symptoms of Varicose Eczema. These sensations can vary in intensity but are typically more pronounced when the condition is exacerbated. Here's a closer look at these symptoms:

Itching Pruritus: Intense itching is a characteristic feature of Varicose Eczema. The itchiness can be relentless and may

Varicose eczema Complete treatment

interfere with daily activities and sleep. Scratching the itchy skin can further damage the skin barrier, making it susceptible to infections.

Discomfort and Pain: Many individuals with Varicose Eczema experience discomfort, aching, or a heavy feeling in their legs, especially after prolonged periods of standing or sitting. Some may also experience a burning or throbbing sensation. This discomfort can impact mobility and overall quality of life.

Potential Complications

Varicose Eczema, if left untreated or poorly managed, can lead to several potential complications, some of which can be severe. It's crucial to be aware of these complications and seek medical attention if you suspect any of them:

Skin Ulcers-Venous Ulcers: Prolonged inflammation and skin changes can progress to the development of open sores or

Varicose eczema Complete treatment

ulcers, typically in the lower leg or ankle area. Venous ulcers are painful, slow to heal, and can become infected.

Cellulitis: The compromised skin barrier in Varicose Eczema increases the risk of bacterial infections like cellulitis. Cellulitis is characterized by redness, warmth, swelling, and tenderness in the affected area. It requires prompt treatment with antibiotics.

Deep Vein Thrombosis DVT: Although less common, severe venous insufficiency associated with Varicose Eczema can increase the risk of blood clots in the deep veins of the legs. DVT is a serious condition that requires immediate medical attention, as it can lead to pulmonary embolism a clot traveling to the lungs.

Eczema Herpeticum: In rare cases, Varicose Eczema can be complicated by a viral skin infection called eczema herpeticum, typically caused by the herpes simplex virus. This requires antiviral treatment.

Skin Atrophy: Prolonged inflammation and use of topical steroids to manage symptoms can lead to thinning of the skin skin atrophy.

Varicose eczema Complete treatment

Understanding these potential complications underscores the importance of early diagnosis and effective management of Varicose Eczema. Timely medical intervention can help prevent or mitigate these issues, improving the overall prognosis for individuals with this condition.

CHAPTER 3

DIAGNOSIS

Diagnosing Varicose Eczema typically involves a combination of clinical evaluation, medical history, and specialized tests. The primary goal is to identify the presence of underlying chronic venous insufficiency, which is causing the skin changes and symptoms associated with Varicose Eczema.

Varicose eczema Complete treatment

Medical History and Physical Examination

Medical History: The diagnostic process often begins with a comprehensive medical history. The healthcare provider will inquire about the patient's symptoms, including when they started, their severity, and any factors that worsen or alleviate them. Additionally, the patient's overall health and any preexisting medical conditions are discussed.

Physical Examination: A thorough physical examination is crucial for diagnosing Varicose Eczema. During this examination, the healthcare provider will closely inspect the affected areas, typically the lower legs and ankles. They will look for characteristic signs, including skin discoloration, thickening, scaling, and varicose veins. Palpation of the legs can help identify areas of tenderness or swelling. The presence of open sores or ulcers may also be assessed.

Doppler Ultrasound

Purpose: Doppler ultrasound is a key diagnostic tool for Varicose Eczema as it allows for a detailed assessment of the

Varicose eczema Complete treatment

blood flow in the leg veins. It helps identify underlying venous insufficiency, which is often the root cause of the condition.

Procedure: During a Doppler ultrasound, a handheld device emitting high-frequency sound waves (ultrasound) is used to create images of the leg veins and assess the direction and speed of blood flow. It can detect blood clots, valve dysfunction, and areas of reflux where blood flows backward instead of toward the heart.

Results: The results of a Doppler ultrasound provide essential information about the status of the veins in the legs. If venous insufficiency is confirmed, it helps guide treatment decisions, such as whether compression therapy or a medical procedure is necessary.

Other Diagnostic Tests

In some cases, additional diagnostic tests may be ordered to further evaluate the condition and rule out other potential causes of skin symptoms. These tests may include:

Duplex Ultrasound: This is an advanced form of Doppler ultrasound that combines traditional ultrasound with color Doppler imaging. It provides detailed visualizations of the veins and blood flow patterns, aiding in the assessment of venous insufficiency.

CT or MRI Scans: While less commonly used, computed tomography C.T or magnetic resonance imaging M.R.I scans may be employed to visualize the veins and identify any structural abnormalities or blood clots.

Skin Biopsy: In rare cases where the diagnosis is uncertain or other skin conditions are suspected, a skin biopsy may be performed. A small sample of skin is removed and examined under a microscope to assess the presence of inflammation or other skin disorders.

Varicose eczema Complete treatment

The combination of medical history, physical examination, and specialized tests like Doppler ultrasound is essential for accurately diagnosing Varicose Eczema and determining the most appropriate treatment approach. Early and precise diagnosis is crucial for effective management and preventing complications associated with this condition.

CHAPTER 4

TREATMENT OPTIONS

the various treatment options for Varicose Eczema, including lifestyle changes, topical medications, compression therapy, medications, and procedures/surgery

The management of Varicose Eczema aims to alleviate symptoms, improve the appearance of the skin, and address the underlying venous insufficiency. The choice of treatment depends on the severity of the condition and may involve a combination of the following approaches:

Varicose eczema Complete treatment

Lifestyle Changes

Elevation: Elevating the affected leg(s) whenever possible, especially when resting or sleeping, can help reduce swelling and improve blood flow. Keeping the legs elevated above heart level is particularly effective.

Regular Exercise: Engaging in regular low-impact exercises, such as walking or swimming, can promote healthy circulation. These exercises also help strengthen the leg muscles, which can assist in pumping blood back to the heart.

Weight Management: Maintaining a healthy weight can reduce the pressure on the leg veins, which is especially important if excess weight contributes to venous insufficiency.

Avoiding Prolonged Standing or Sitting: If possible, avoid long periods of standing or sitting. If prolonged sitting is necessary, taking breaks to walk and stretch can help.

Compression Stockings: Wearing graduated compression stockings, as prescribed by a healthcare provider, can help improve venous return by providing external pressure to support proper blood flow.

Topical Medications

Emollients: Emollient creams or ointments are often recommended to keep the skin moisturized and prevent dryness and flakiness.

Topical Steroids: For managing inflammation and itching, topical steroids may be prescribed in mild to moderate cases. These should be used under medical supervision and for limited durations to avoid potential side effects.

Topical Calcineurin Inhibitors: In some cases, healthcare providers may recommend non-steroidal topical treatments like calcineurin inhibitors to control inflammation and itching.

Varicose eczema Complete treatment

Compression Therapy

Compression Stockings: Graduated compression stockings are designed to apply pressure from the ankle up the leg, gradually decreasing in pressure as they move higher. This helps improve venous return and reduces swelling. Proper fitting and prescription are essential to ensure effectiveness.

Unna Boot: In more severe cases or when ulcers are present, an Unna boot a special bandage containing zinc oxide paste may be applied to the affected leg to promote healing and reduce inflammation.

Medications

Oral Medications: In certain situations, oral medications such as diuretics may be prescribed to reduce fluid retention and swelling.

Varicose eczema Complete treatment

Antibiotics: If there is evidence of infection, antibiotics may be necessary to treat or prevent further complications.

Procedures and Surgery

Endovenous Laser Ablation E.V.L.A: EVLA is a minimally invasive procedure that uses laser energy to seal off problematic veins, redirecting blood flow to healthier veins. This can effectively treat underlying venous insufficiency.

Radiofrequency Ablation RFA: Similar to EVLA, RFA uses radiofrequency energy to close off malfunctioning veins.

Sclerotherapy: This procedure involves injecting a sclerosing agent into varicose veins, causing them to collapse and eventually be reabsorbed by the body.

Vein Stripping: In cases where varicose veins are extensive and causing significant symptoms, vein stripping surgery may be considered. This involves removing the affected veins through small incisions.

Skin Grafting or Flap Surgery: If skin ulcers have developed, surgical techniques like grafting or flap surgery may be necessary to promote wound healing.

The choice of treatment depends on the individual's specific condition and the severity of Varicose Eczema. Healthcare providers will tailor the treatment plan to address both the skin symptoms and the underlying venous insufficiency, with the goal of improving overall quality of life and preventing complications. It's important for individuals with Varicose Eczema to work closely with their healthcare team to determine the most suitable approach.

CHAPTER 5

PREVENTION AND SELF-CARE

prevention and self-care strategies for Varicose Eczema, which can help manage symptoms and reduce the risk of complications.

Varicose eczema Complete treatment

Preventing Varicose Eczema and managing its symptoms often involve a combination of lifestyle changes and self-care practices. These strategies aim to improve circulation, protect the skin, and minimize the impact of venous insufficiency. Here are key components of prevention and self-care:

Maintaining Healthy Leg Circulation

Exercise Regularly: Engage in regular physical activity that promotes leg muscle strength and circulation. Activities like walking, swimming, and cycling are excellent choices. These exercises help pump blood from the legs back to the heart.

Avoid Prolonged Sitting or Standing: If your work or lifestyle involves long periods of sitting or standing, take breaks to move and elevate your legs when possible. Simple leg stretches and ankle pumps can help prevent blood from pooling in the lower limbs.

Elevate Your Legs: Elevating your legs above heart level when resting can aid in reducing swelling and improving blood flow. Ideally, do this for 15-30 minutes several times a day.

Varicose eczema Complete treatment

Maintain a Healthy Weight: Excess body weight can increase pressure on the leg veins, exacerbating venous insufficiency. Managing your weight through a balanced diet and regular exercise is beneficial.

Skin Care Tips

Keep Skin Moisturized: Apply emollient creams or ointments regularly to maintain skin moisture and reduce dryness. This can help prevent scaling and flakiness.

Avoid Harsh Soaps: Use mild, fragrance-free soaps and avoid hot baths or showers, as hot water can further dry out the skin.

Pat, Don't Rub: After bathing or showering, gently pat your skin dry with a soft towel rather than rubbing vigorously.

Wear Loose-Fitting Clothing: Choose loose-fitting clothing to avoid constriction of blood flow. Tight clothing can worsen venous insufficiency.

Protect Skin from Sun: Excessive sun exposure can damage already sensitive skin. Use sunscreen and wear protective clothing, especially if you have skin discoloration or hyperpigmentation.

Lifestyle Modifications

Diet: A diet rich in fiber, antioxidants, and anti-inflammatory foods may help support vascular health. This includes fruits, vegetables, whole grains, and foods high in omega-3 fatty acids like fatty fish.

Hydration: Stay well-hydrated to maintain blood volume and circulation. Adequate hydration can help prevent blood from becoming too viscous.

Avoid Smoking: Smoking can damage blood vessels and worsen circulation problems. If you smoke, consider quitting.

Compression Stockings: If prescribed by a healthcare provider, wear graduated compression stockings regularly. These provide external pressure to support blood flow.

Varicose eczema Complete treatment

Manage Underlying Conditions: If you have underlying conditions like hypertension or diabetes, managing them effectively can contribute to overall vascular health.

Consult with Specialists: Regular check-ups with vascular specialists and dermatologists can help monitor your condition and ensure that you are following the best preventive and self-care practices.

Prevention and self-care are crucial aspects of managing Varicose Eczema. While these strategies can help alleviate symptoms and reduce the risk of complications, it's important to work closely with healthcare professionals to tailor a plan that meets your specific needs and addresses any underlying venous insufficiency.

CHAPTER 6

LIVING WITH VARICOSE ECZEMA

Varicose eczema Complete treatment

Living with Varicose Eczema can be challenging, as it often involves chronic symptoms that affect both the physical and emotional well-being of individuals. However, with proper management and self-care, many people can lead fulfilling lives while minimizing the impact of this condition.

Coping with Symptoms

Itching Management: Since itching is a common and distressing symptom, it's essential to employ strategies to alleviate it. This can include using prescribed topical treatments, keeping the skin moisturized, and avoiding scratching. Wearing loose-fitting clothing made of breathable fabrics can also help reduce irritation.

Pain and Discomfort: For those experiencing pain and discomfort, elevation of the legs can provide relief. Over-the-counter pain relievers, as recommended by a healthcare provider, can be used for mild pain. More severe discomfort may require prescription medications or other interventions.

Varicose eczema Complete treatment

Skin Care: Maintaining a consistent skincare routine is crucial. Use mild soaps, moisturizers, and sunscreen to protect the skin. Avoid harsh or fragranced products that can exacerbate skin sensitivity.

Emotional Well-being: Coping with a chronic skin condition like Varicose Eczema can have emotional and psychological effects. It's essential to seek emotional support from friends, family, or mental health professionals if needed. Support groups or counseling can provide a safe space to discuss concerns and share experiences with others facing similar challenges.

Monitoring and Follow-up

Regular Check-ups: Individuals with Varicose Eczema should schedule regular follow-up appointments with their healthcare providers. These appointments allow for monitoring of the condition's progress, evaluation of treatment effectiveness, and adjustments to the treatment plan as needed.

Assessing Complications: It's crucial to be vigilant for any signs of complications, such as skin ulcers or infections. Early

Varicose eczema Complete treatment

detection and treatment of these complications can prevent them from worsening.

Medication Review: If prescribed medications are part of the treatment plan, discuss their effectiveness and any potential side effects with your healthcare provider during follow-up visits.

Support and Resources

Patient Support Groups: Joining patient support groups or online forums dedicated to Varicose Eczema can provide a sense of community and a platform to exchange information and experiences. Connecting with others who understand the challenges of living with the condition can be comforting and empowering.

Educational Resources: Seek reliable sources of information about Varicose Eczema, its treatment, and self-care practices.

Consult medical literature, reputable websites, and educational materials provided by healthcare professionals.

Healthcare Team: Maintain open communication with your healthcare team, which may include dermatologists, vascular specialists, and wound care specialists. Ask questions and voice any concerns you have about your condition, treatment, or self-care routines.

Insurance and Financial Support: If your Varicose Eczema treatment involves ongoing medical expenses, explore your health insurance coverage and inquire about available financial assistance or support programs.

Living with Varicose Eczema is manageable with proper care, support, and the guidance of healthcare professionals. By taking a proactive approach to symptom management, staying informed, and seeking support when needed, individuals can improve their quality of life while effectively managing this condition.

CONCLUSION

In conclusion, Varicose Eczema, also known as stasis dermatitis, is a skin condition closely tied to underlying circulatory issues, specifically chronic venous insufficiency. It manifests as skin changes, itching, discomfort, and, in severe cases, can lead to complications like skin ulcers and infections. While living with Varicose Eczema can pose challenges, there are numerous strategies and treatments available to manage this condition effectively and improve one's quality of life.

Summary of Varicose Eczema

Varicose Eczema is characterized by skin discoloration, dryness, scaling, itching, and discomfort, primarily affecting the lower legs and ankles. It is a secondary skin condition resulting from chronic venous insufficiency, which causes blood to pool in the leg veins. Over time, this condition can lead to varicose veins and skin changes. Varicose Eczema can be diagnosed through medical history, physical examination, Doppler ultrasound, and other diagnostic tests. Treatment options include lifestyle changes, topical medications, compression therapy, medications, and procedures/surgery.

Varicose eczema Complete treatment

Importance of Early Detection and Management

Early detection and management of Varicose Eczema are of paramount importance for several reasons:

Preventing Complications: Early intervention can prevent the development of complications such as skin ulcers, cellulitis, and deep vein thrombosis DVT. These complications can be severe and challenging to treat, making prevention a top priority.

Symptom Relief: Timely treatment can alleviate the distressing symptoms of Varicose Eczema, including itching, pain, and discomfort. This significantly improves the individual's quality of life and overall well-being.

Minimizing Skin Changes: Addressing Varicose Eczema early can help minimize skin changes and discoloration, preserving the appearance of the affected area.

Managing Underlying Causes: By identifying and managing the underlying circulatory issues, such as venous insufficiency, early

Varicose eczema Complete treatment

intervention can potentially halt or slow down the progression of the condition, preventing further damage to the veins and skin.

Improved Outcomes: The earlier Varicose Eczema is diagnosed and treated, the better the chances of successful outcomes. Effective management can help individuals lead active and fulfilling lives with minimal disruption.

In essence, early detection and proactive management of Varicose Eczema are key to maintaining skin health, preventing complications, and optimizing the overall quality of life for individuals affected by this condition. Regular medical check-ups, adherence to treatment plans, and lifestyle adjustments can make a significant difference in managing and living with Varicose Eczema.

Varicose eczema Complete treatment